Low Carb Baker

Table of content

Book 1

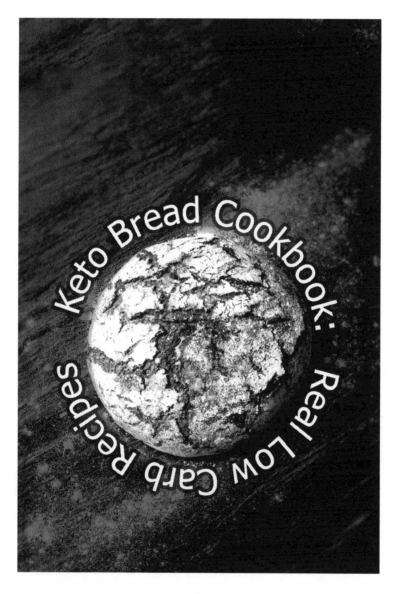

Keto Bread Cookbook: Real Low Carb Recipes

Keto Bread Cookbook:

Real Low Carb Recipes

Introduction

You may well have heard of the Keto diet already. It is even possible that you have dismissed it as yet another diet fad. However, the Keto diet is based on science and a good understanding of the human body. This type of diet has been an option for many years; it has often been referred to as simply the low carb diet or sometimes even the low carb, high fat (LCHF) diet. The fact is that it involves changing your approach to eating either temporarily or permanently. Doing so has been noted to provide an array of benefits.

Research suggests that a Keto diet can assist with controlling epilepsy, a reduction n the risk of contracting Alzheimer's, Parkinson's and even cancer. It can also be an effective way to lose weight whilst improving your energy levels and mental abilities!

The body generally creates energy by converting all the carbohydrates you consume into insulin and glucose. The insulin carries the glucose around the body; allowing it to reach every muscle and organ where it is burnt as a fuel. The modern diet is packed full of carbohydrates; they are in processed foods; particularly starchy foods such as bread, potatoes and even pasta. Many advocates of this diet will place the emphasis of their food habits on eating a high fat, low carb and even low protein diet. However, what is really important is reducing your carbohydrate intake. In general you will need to consume less than fifty grams of carbs a day, although a maximum of twenty is considered more effective.

Once you reduce your carb intake sufficiently your body will need to find an alternative source of energy. It enters what is known as ketosis. At this point the liver converts fat into ketones. These ketones can be burnt by the body in the same way that glucose is. The main difference is that these provide a steady supply of energy rather than sudden hits. Although it can be difficult to transition to a new diet; this is worthwhile! For as long as you keep your body in a state of ketosis you will be burning fat and not glucose. This will often quickly affect the shape of your body as you consume the excess fat and lose weight.

Unfortunately, many traditional recipes rely on flour to bind the ingredients together. This is not an option on the keto diet and substitute options; such as almond flour, do not have the same effect. Many items on this diet can struggle to bind or, b y combining the right ingredients, can manage to bind but end up being too sticky. Getting the recipe right is crucial to creating delicious and wholesome alternatives to the traditional calorie rich foods. This book will provide you with a range of recipes to try and be impressed by.

It is important to note that the Keto diet is not for everyone. It is particularly important to get medical advice if you are already taking prescription medicine.

Chapter 1 – Bread; the Staple of Life

Bread is possibly one of the most popular and common items eaten around the world. It can be used to make a sandwich, add flavor and texture to a meal or simply to fill you up between meals.

Once you start looking at bread you will realize that there are many different options; ranging from sliced loafs to baguettes and even flat breads. It is also worth noting that many mass produced breads are not just a rich source of carbohydrates; they often have vitamins added. B1 is one of the most common although there is some vitamin A, R, K and even vitamin D. Bread is also an excellent convenience food; it is generally possible to take it anywhere with you.

Bread is impressive as it appears in a huge range of guises: virtually all shapes and sizes can and are produced. It can fulfill a variety of roles in your diet. It is interesting to note that the majority of recipes which are designed to encourage ketosis are also excellent choices for anyone with a glucose tolerance issue. The issue is, as bread is often used to fill a gap in your diet, how can you ensure your body is getting all the nutrients it needs without consuming this high calorie option. The answer lies in the following recipes where you can discover delicious, healthy alternatives which are low in carbohydrates and will boost your ability to get things done!

1. *Egg Bread Buns*

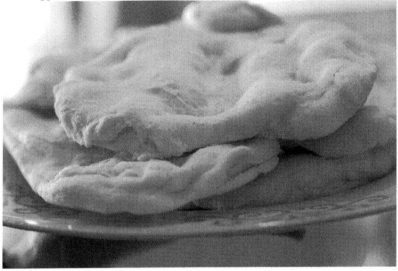

Photo made by: Kent Goldman

This bread is usually crafted as a roll and has almost no carbs in it. The fact that they are flourless means that they are acceptable by those with gluten intolerance. They are surprising easy to make and delicious.

In fact this bread is similar in nature to a normal bun; you can even choose to use them as part of a savory dish or a sweet one!

Ingredients:

3 Large eggs

¼ tsp Cream of tartar

100g Cream Cheese

Pinch of salt

You will need to separate the whites from the yolks of your eggs. The whites should be placed in a bowl and whisked with the cream of tartar until the mixture is thick. Separately you will need to whisk the yolks, full fat cream cheese and a pinch of salt. This should be mixed until smooth.

You can then fold your egg whites into the other mixture. It is important to fold and not stir as this will keep the air trapped in the mixture. You must repeat the folding process until it is all blended.

Finally, place six mounds onto a baking sheet and put in a pre-heated oven at 300 Fahrenheit for approximately thirty minutes.

Nutrient Information

The recipe is designed to make four buns. Each has ninety calories, eight grams of fat and less than one of carbohydrates, sodium, fiber and protein

2. *Sugar Free Corn bread*

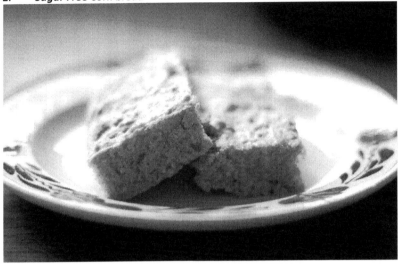

Photo made by: Suzette

Sugar is something which is best reduced on any kind of diet. It can be used immediately by the body to create energy; in the same way that glucose is. Consuming more than a little sugar will take you out of the ketosis state and start to reverse the good effects you are having on your body. This recipe is an excellent alternative.

Ingredients

2 Cups Almond Meal

¼ cup sweetener

1 tsp salt

4 tsp baking powder

2 eggs

½ cup vanilla almond milk

1/3 cup coconut oil

15oz baby corn – this part is optional.

Start by mixing the almond meal, sweetener, salt and baking powder. Separately break the eggs in a bowl and whisk them smooth. To the eggs add the vanilla almond milk and a third of a cup of coconut milk. The slowly blend the two mixtures together until thoroughly mixed and smooth.

The mixture can then be placed on a greased or lined baking tray and cooked for twenty five minutes at 350 Fahrenheit. Slice according to need and enjoy!

Nutritional Info

Each corn bread provides roughly 173 calories, 5g carbohydrates, 18g fat and 4.5g protein.

3.   *Coconut and Almond Bread*
Impressively you may find it difficult to tell the difference between this natural bread and the one you are accustomed to and used to purchase from the shops regularly. It is excellent for toast or sandwiches. Try it with an egg on top to get you fired up for the day!

Ingredients

1 ½ Cups almond flour

2 tbsp coconut flour

¼ cup flaxseed meal

Pinch of salt

1 ½ tsp baking soda

5 eggs

¼ cup coconut oil

1 tsp sweetener

1 tbsp cider vinegar

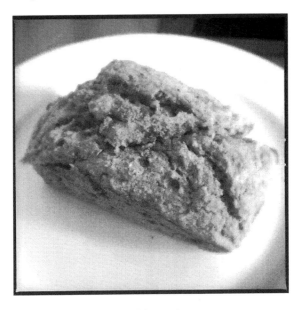

Photo made by: Ryan Ruppe

Mix the almond flour, coconut flour, flax, salt and the baking soda in a bowl. You can even do this bit in a food processor. Once all the ingredients are merged add the vinegar, eggs and oil and continue mixing.

Then pour the mix into a prepared loaf tin and cook for thirty minutes on 350 Fahrenheit. It is ready as soon as it has left the oven.

Nutrition

Assuming you cut this into eight slices each one will have approximately 267 calories, 3g net carbs, 24g fat and 9g protein.

4.   *Flax Bread*

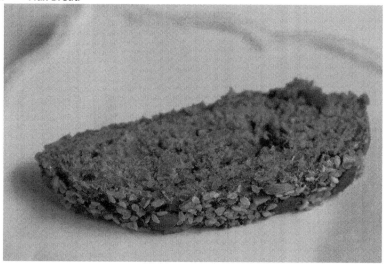

Photo made by: veganbaking.net

This is often referred to as focaccia type bread simple because it is cooked flat on a baking tray; similar to the way focaccia is made. It is very versatile bread which can be used as toast or for sandwiches.

Ingredients

2 cups flax meal

1 tbsp baking powder

Pinch of salt

2 Tbsp sweetener

5 Eggs – these will need to be beaten.

½ cup water.

A little oil

Start by mixing the flax meal, baking powder, salt and sweetener in a bowl. Once thoroughly combined add the eggs, water and a little oil. It is important to make sure this is mixed thoroughly. It will then need to be left for several minutes before being poured into a baking tray; keeping an eye on the thickness of the mix. It needs to be cooked on 350 Fahrenheit for twenty five minutes and then left to cool. Then you can cut and consume to your heart's content.

Nutrition

Each bread should make approximately twelve slices with just under a gram of carbohydrates in each! There is also 6g protein and 185 calories.

5.   *Almond Faux Buns*

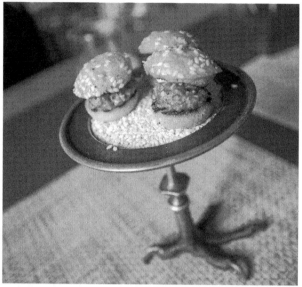

Photo made by: <u>City Foodsters</u>

This creates a perfect burger bap or opportunity for a delicious sandwich without the carbs. Just the sight of the bun will start you thinking about what you can put with it!

Ingredients

1 Cup Almond Flour

2 tsp baking powder

2 large eggs

5 tbsp butter – this will need to be melted.

Mix the almond flour with the baking powder. You can then whisk the two large eggs separately and add the melted butter. Mix this with the dry ingredients to create your dough. Now split the mixture into six muffin size shapes on a baking tray. If you prefer, you can use a muffin pan to create several buns. Finally they should be cooked for fifteen minutes at 350 Fahrenheit. Ideally the finished bread should be left to cool on a wire rack.

Nutrition

This recipe makes two of these faux buns, which will provide 35 grams of fat, 7 of carbohydrates, 3 grams of fiber, 10 grams of protein and 373 calories.

6.   *Garlic Bread with Cheese*

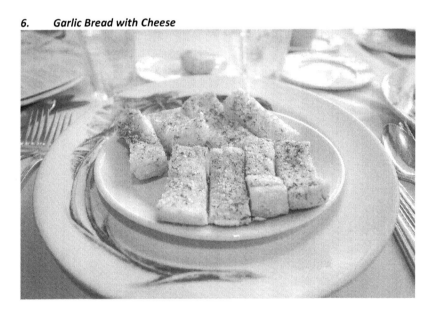

Photo made by: City Foodsters

Almost everyone loves garlic bread, especially if it is dripping with cheese! However, adhering to a keto diet means being unable to eat the garlic bread you would normally buy in the shops. Fortunately there is a delicious alternative which is just as easy to make and tastes just as good.

Ingredients

¼ cup almond flour

1 tbsp coconut flour

Pinch of salt

Pinch of garlic powder

¼ cup warm water

1 tsp coconut sugar

1tsp yeast

3 large egg whites

½ cup grated mozzarella

Start by mixing the almond flour with the coconut flour, salt and garlic powder. Once this is thoroughly mixed up you can put it to one side.

Next in a separate bowl you should mix the warm water with the coconut sugar and yeast. Let this mixture stand for two minutes before mixing both lots together. You will also need to put in two tablespoons of olive oil.

Finally, add the three beaten egg whites and the half a cup of grated mozzarella. You can then pour the mixture onto a baking tray and cook. It should take just fifteen minutes at 400 Fahrenheit.

Whilst you are waiting you will need to merge two tablespoon of butter with a little garlic powder and a pinch of salt. When the bread is ready spread this mixture across the bread and return to the oven for another ten minutes.

Nutrition

The recipe should cut into ten pieces; each peace will have 175 calories, 2g net carbs, 16 grams of fat and eight grams of protein.

Chapter 2 – The Art of Keto Flat Bread

Flat breads are incredibly versatile and delicious to eat; even in their Keto state! There are excellent for using as pizza bases, making tasty sandwiches with or even adding ingredients to and simply enjoying as they are. Flat breads offer a nice change to the more traditional style breads and can actually taste superior as well.

In general this type of bread is easy to make and cook; they can be enjoyed warm or cold and at any time of the day!

1.   *Soy Flat Bread*

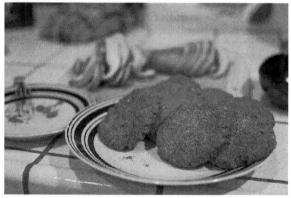

Photo made by: Zach Zupancic

It may be obvious but this bread is designed to be made with soy flour instead of the usual wheat flour. Not only does this reduce the number of carbs in the bread it also makes it an acceptable choice for anyone with a gluten allergy. The recipe can be mixed by hand but you will generally find a more positive effect is produced by using an electric food processor. This will blend the ingredients more finely whilst preserving the air in the mixture.

Ingredients

1 ¼ cups Soy Flour

2 tsp Baking Powder

Pinch of salt

1 Tbsp onion powder

1 Tbsp garlic powder – optional

1 cup warm water

Start by mixing the soy flour with the baking powder and a large pinch of the salt. You can then add onion powder and garlic powder. If you prefer you can reduce the amounts of these or even leave one of them out. The electric food processor should have it perfectly blended within a minute or two.

Next you should keep the mixer going and slowly add one cup of warm water. The dough will become sticky which is exactly how you want it!

Lightly dust your hands with soy flour before rolling the dough into a ball and take small fist sizes of the dough. These should be gently rolled into circles and then lightly fried in olive oil until golden brown. It should not take more than two or three minutes per side. It is advisable to consume the flat breads within an hour of having made them. Alternatively you can store the dough in a fridge for one week and make them as you need or want them.

Nutrition

This recipe should make eight flat breads. Each one will have 118 calories, 9.7 g fats, 4.4 g carbohydrate and 5.1 g protein.

2.   *Coconut Psyllium Flat Bread*

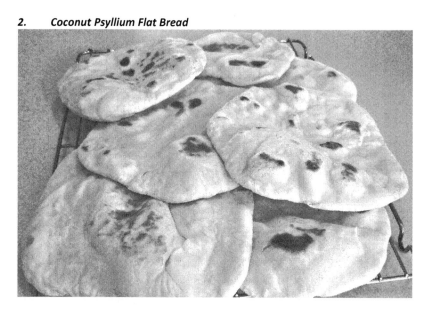

This flat bread has a delightful light yet filling texture and is exceptionally good with a sweet topping; such as fresh berries.

Ingredients

60 grams coconut flour

2 Tbsp Psyllium husk powder

Salt

1 tsp Baking powder

Mixed herbs

40 grams coconut oil

200 grams water

Firstly place 60 grams of coconut flour in a bowl and add the psyllium husk powder. Blend them thoroughly before adding a large pinch of salt and the baking powder. Whilst mixing all these ingredients you can sprinkle in your favorite spices or herbs to add a little extra zing to your flat bread; don't be afraid to experiment!

You will then need to add the coconut oil and continue to mix thoroughly. The mixture should start to look buttery. Slowly add the water, stirring consistently. The mixture will become dough like; if it has reached the required consistency before you have added all the water then do not add the last bit! Ideally it should be divided into three and each part should be flattened before being placed on a baking tray; preferably on grease proof paper.

Each of the flat breads should be cooked in a frying pan with a little olive oil or coconut oil. It should take no more than three minutes per side to ensure they look and taste fantastic.

Nutrition

Each one will have approximately 185 calories, 12g fat, 3g protein, 16g carbohydrates and 11g fiber; giving a net carb intake of 5g.

3.   *Simple Flat Bread*

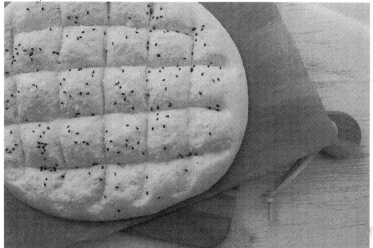

Sometimes you need a really simple and quick recipe; especially if you have had a long day at the office. The temptation will be to grab some convenience food which will ruin the efforts you have been making to adhere to the Keto diet. Instead of succumbing to temptation, try one making this quick and easy flat bread. It can accompany almost any meal or the recipe can be tweaked to provide a wholesome meal in itself.

Ingredients

145g almond flour

30g Flax seed

Salt

2 Large eggs

120ml Heavy cream

Mix together all the ingredients! This includes the almond flour, flaxseed, a large pinch of salt, 2 large eggs and the heavy cream. You can do this by hand with a whisk or in a food processor. After a few minutes it should be smooth and have the appearance of pancake batter.

To cook it you will need to pour the mixture onto a baking tray which has been lined with baking paper. To get the best results ensure your mixture is no thicker than 1cm. It will need approximately twenty five minutes at 300 Fahrenheit. Allow to cool for ten minutes before adding toppings, eating as is or even creating a sandwich!

Nutrition

These figures are for the entire mixture; 1609 calories, 13 g carbs, 145g fat and 59g protein. You will get between eight and sixteen slices and can calculate the actual values accordingly.

4. *Parmesan Flat Bread*

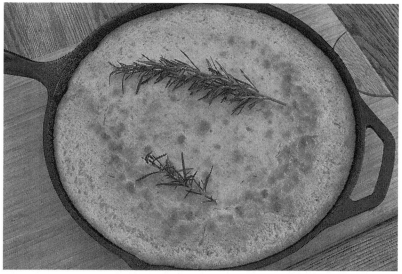

Photo made by: jeffreyw

This is an excellent example of adding a little variance to an otherwise extremely simple recipe. The result is a delicious flat bread which can accompany your meal or be a meal in itself! If parmesan is not your preferred choice then it can be replaced with any other similar hard cheese.

Ingredients

½ cup parmesan cheese; grated

3 cloves garlic

Black pepper

3 large eggs

¼ cup coconut flour

Place the parmesan cheese into a bowl and add the cloves of garlic. These should already have been finely minced. Mix, the ingredients together along with a large pinch of black pepper; you can also add salt if you wish.

Once they have all been combined properly it is time to add the three large eggs. However, it is essential to add them one at a time; ensuring each one is completed absorbed by the mixture before moving onto the next. You can then add the coconut flour. Again this will need to be done slowly and carefully to ensure it is fully absorbed. It is advisable to leave the combined mixture sitting in the bowl for several minutes before you take the next step.

Once you are ready, pour the complete mixture into a lined baking tray and put it in the oven. It will take approximately twenty minutes at 375 Fahrenheit. After it has been in fifteen minutes it can be removed and some extra cheese should be sprinkled on top before it is returned to the cooker for a further five minutes. This will allow the cheese to melt into the flat bread and ensure it tastes fantastic!

Nutrition

The complete recipe has the following values. You can work out approximate values for the amount you eat depending upon how many it cuts into.

297 calories, 12g fat, 15g protein and 3g net carbs.

5. The Keto Naan

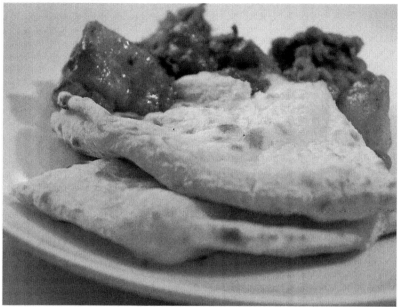

Naan breads are a traditional accompaniment to a curry but you can also use them to make sandwiches or simply add a few extra spices and eat them by themselves.

Ingredients

½ cup coconut flour

1 Tbsp psyllium husk powder

Salt

1 cup hot water

This is an incredible quick and easy bread to make. Start by heating up you cup of water until it is nearly boiling. Whilst it is warming mix the coconut flour and psyllium husk powder in a bowl with one or two pinches of salt; to your preferred taste. You can also choose to add pepper, garlic powder, onion powder or any mixture of herbs and spices you like.

You will now be able to slowly add the hot water, stirring as you go. The mixture will gradually become dough like. Once completed it is best to leave the mixture for five minutes; ideally in the fridge. This will firm it slightly and make it easier to manage when creating your naan's.

When ready, form seven balls from your dough mixture and roll each one of them out. Once they are flat you can place them on a baking tray. You may find it is easier to roll them between two bits of baking paper; it depends upon how sticky they are to the touch. You can then slide the tray into the oven at 350 Fahrenheit. Cook for roughly ten minutes before turning them all over and cooking for a further ten minutes. They can be eaten immediately or will keep for a while if required.

Nutrition

Assuming you have made seven naan's from this recipe, each one will have approximately 35 calories, 1.2g fat, 1.7g net carbs and 1.3g protein. Filling and healthy!

6. Coconut Flour Flatbread

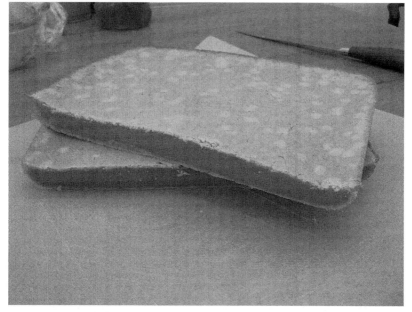

Photo made by: stu_spivack

This is one of the first recipes that many people try when attempting flat bread or even more conventional breads in-line with the keto lifestyle. It is easy to make and, if done properly, can taste fantastic. Sometimes simple is best!

Ingredients

1 Tbsp Coconut flour

1 Large egg

1 Tbsp parmesan cheese

Baking soda

Baking Powder

Salt

Mixed Herbs

Milk

Simply combine all the ingredients, except the parmesan cheese, in a bowl. You should use a large pinch of salt, baking soda and the baking powder. The mixed herbs are an optional addition. You can select your own flavors! You will need to stir thoroughly; you may prefer to use an electric whisk or blender.

Once it is smooth and batter like you will be able to heat a little oil in a pan and then add two circles of the batter; roughly the same size. Cook them for several minutes before flipping them. Ideally the top should be bubbling indicating the bottom has browned off. Once you have flipped them you can add your parmesan on top of the flat bread. Alternatively you can use a different type of cheese. Place the second flat bread on top and continue cooking until the inside has melted. You will then need to repeat the process. This mixture should provide you with two 'sandwiches'.

Nutrition

Based on you making two sandwiches, the nutritional information per sandwich would be; 103 calories, 4g protein, 8g fat and 2g net carbs.

Chapter 3 – Additional Bread Ideas for the Keto Enthusiast

The keto lifestyle requires dedication and, just like any dietary plan, a commitment to the key ingredients. This can be made much easier if you have an extensive selection of recipes to choose from. After all, they say variety is the spice of life! The following recipes are all acceptable on the keto diet and can add that all important variance:

1. The Baguette

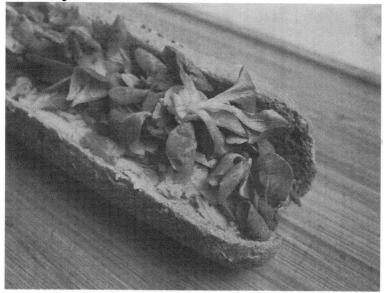

This is one of the traditional ways to make a delicious lunchtime snack. It is also one of the most difficult to create when living on a keto diet or even a gluten free one. Fortunately this recipe manages to achieve this and provides you with a sandwich size baguette which is little different from the traditional versions.

Ingredients

1 ½ cup almond flour

5 Tbsp psyllium husk powder

3 egg whites

2 ½ Tbsp cider vinegar

1 cup boiling water

Baking Powder

Salt

You will need to start by mixing the almond flour with the psyllium husk powder and two teaspoons of baking powder. You can also add a pinch of salt, if required. You have managed to mix these up thoroughly you can add the egg whites and the cider vinegar. Continue to mix and you will see a thick dough is forming. This can be turned into a normal dough by adding the boiling water. It is important to do this slowly as you may find that just under a cup is enough to create the right dough.

You can then create four or five one inch long baguettes. They will grow when cooked. These need to go on a greased or lined baking tray and then into the oven for fifty five minutes at 350 Fahrenheit. You can eat them as soon as they are cooked; just be careful; they will be hot!

Nutrition

This mixture is designed to make five small baguettes. Each one will have approximately 209 calories, 14.2g fat, 8.2g protein and 5.2g net carbs.

2.   *Plain and Simple Almond Flour Bread*

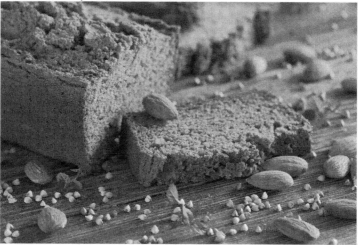

If you crave toast or sandwiches like you use to eat them then this is the recipe for you. It is relatively heavy but holds together in a similar way to traditional bread; making it the perfect choice for a wide variety of sandwiches and other more traditional snacks.

Ingredients

2 ½ cups almond flour

½ cup oat fiber (not oat flour)

¼ cup protein powder

1 Tbsp erythritol

6 oz Greek yoghurt

6Tbsp butter

4 large eggs

6 Tbsp Almond milk

Baking powder

Baking soda

Xanthan gum

Salt

Start by whisking, with a hand or electric whisk, the almond flour, erythritol, oat fiber, protein powder and two teaspoons of baking powder. You will also need to add half a teaspoon of baking soda, one teaspoon of xanthan gum and a pinch of salt.

Once combined set this aside and select a different bowl to beat the yoghurt into the butter. You should get a smooth paste. Then add the eggs, making sure they are fully beaten in. You can now mix the two bowls and continue beating as you add the almond milk.

Once properly combined pour the mixture into a loaf tin and place in the oven. It should take forty five minute on 325 Fahrenheit. You will need to let it cool in its tin for fifteen minutes before removing and placing on a wire rack. You can then cut and eat at your leisure!

Nutrition

The loaf should cut into fifteen slices. Each slice would have approximately 105 calories, 12g fat, 7g protein and 2.9g net carbs.

3.   *Chia Bread*

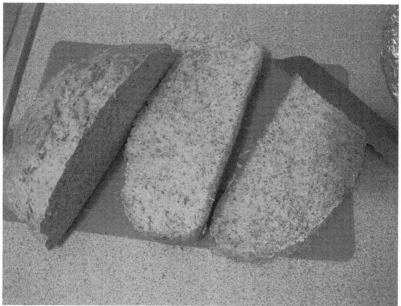

Photo made by: lee leblanc

This is another alternative which is both tasty and holds together very well to make delicious sandwiches.

Ingredients

½ cup coconut flour

1 ¼ cups almond flour

¼ cup chia seeds

5 eggs

1 Tbsp apple cider vinegar

Salt

Baking soda

4 Tbsp coconut oil

Start by mixing the coconut flour with the almond flour, chia seeds, baking soda and a little salt. Separately mix the eggs, vinegar and coconut oil.

Once the ingredients have been mixed fully you can mix the two bowls together; creating a batter like mixture. Simply pour this into a loaf pan and put into the oven for forty five minutes. The temperature will need to be set at 350 Fahrenheit. It is advisable to let it cool before slicing or it will not slice well!

Nutrition

Assuming this loaf is cut into fifteen slices each one would have the following; 133 calories, 11g fat, 5g protein and 3g net carbs.

4.   *The Breakfast Muffin*

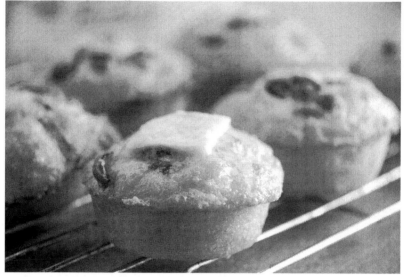

Photo made by: rpavich

Although this is not strictly speaking bread it is an excellent alternative for anyone craving a bacon and egg breakfast or simply looking for a change from the norm. The muffin can be eaten for breakfast or at any time of the day!

Ingredients

120g Chopped Bacon

1 ½ Cups almond flour

Baking powder

Baking soda

½ cup milk

5 tsp sour cream

1 large egg

2 Tbsp butter

Salt

Firstly fry your bacon; it is best if you have chopped it into very small pieces. It should go light brown within a couple of minutes. You can then put the bacon onto a paper towel; this will absorb any excess fat.

Now mix together the almond flour, a teaspoon of baking powder and a large pinch of baking soda. In a separate bowl you can combine the milk, a pinch of salt, the sour cream, egg and the softened or even melted butter. Once both bowls are mixed thoroughly, you can merge them to make one.

You can now add the cooked bacon and a cup of grated parmesan cheese into your mixture. Then put a little of the mix into four molds; next, carefully break one egg into each muffin mold before covering the eggs with the rest of the mixture. Then place the tray in the oven and cook for twenty minutes at 350 Fahrenheit.

Nutrition

The mixture should make four muffins; each of them has 132 calories, 7.5g fat, 3.2g carbohydrates and 8g of protein.

Conclusion

You may be choosing to live the keto lifestyle in order to have a healthy, more natural approach to eating and your body. Alternatively it may be an attempt to lose weight or you may even have realized that many keto recipes are acceptable to people suffering from gluten intolerance. Whatever the reason it is highly likely that you will feel the health benefits in the near future.

Although there may be transitional pains as your body adapts to a new way of eating, these are short lived and the long term benefits far outweigh them. There have been several surveys completed which indicate a keto diet can assist with preventing serious illnesses; such as cancer and Alzheimer's. Perhaps more importantly is the increased levels of energy you will have once you commit to the keto diet. Your body will become accustomed to burning fat and will happily continue to do so as there is always a plentiful supply of fat!

There are those who report issues regarding knowing the nutritional values of all the foods they eat. Although many manufacturers are getting better at labeling their products this is not always the case. Fortunately there are many recipe calculators online which can help with the nutritional value of foods and the recipes in this book provide all the information you need.

Bread is a staple requirement for most people, and the variety of recipes displayed within this book show you that there are still plenty of options even on the keto diet. In fact, you will probably find yourself trying more different things than you would ever have imagined if eating traditional bread.

In addition to the inspiration provided here, there are many forums online which will offer support and advice and you travel along the keto diet journey. Indeed, you will soon be eager to share your own experiences and make improvements to these recipes to suit your own tastes!

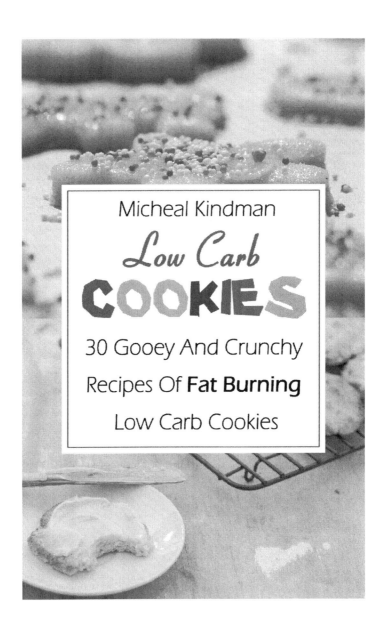

Micheal Kindman

Low Carb

COOKIES

30 Gooey And Crunchy

Recipes Of **Fat Burning**

Low Carb Cookies

Low Carb Cookies
30 Gooey And Crunchy Recipes Of Fat Burning Low Carb Cookies

Cover photo made by: <u>Jules</u>

Introduction

You've been working hard and you've been doing well. You've stuck with your diet though there's been times that it has been purely torture. You've done your research, and you are starting to see the results that you want to see.

But, you can't help but feel deprived. You miss your sweet treats, you miss desserts, and you miss the satisfied feeling of having something that you don't normally get to have. Being low carb may make you feel good most of the time, but you have to admit that there are times when you simply feel deprived.

Thankfully, it doesn't have to be this way – and that is where this book comes in. In it, you are going to discover just how easy it is to eat low carb, enjoy the food you want to enjoy, and still get to have the sweet treats you are craving.

This book is full of recipes that are going to make you feel good, satisfy your sweet tooth, and give you just the fix you were looking for – without making you cheat on your diet. There is no way you can go wrong with these cookies, so don't be afraid to indulge in as many as you want.

Whip up a batch today, and give yourself the reminder of what it's like to indulge in the sweetness of baked goods.

Let's get started.

Chapter 1 – The Recipes

Wonder Cookies

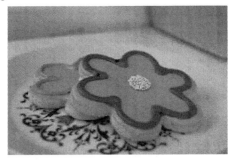

Photo made by: stuart_spivack

Makes: 30

Calories: 36

Carbs: 1g

Fats: 1g

What you will need:

1/3 cup butter

1 oz cream cheese

1/3 cup Swerve Sweetener

1 egg

tsp vanilla extract

1 tsp almond extract

1 cup coconut flour (or half coconut half almond flour)

1 tsp baking powder

pinch of salt

natural food dye

Directions:

Preheat oven to 350 degrees F.

Spray 2 cookie sheets with no stick cooking spray, or line with parchment paper and set aside.

In a large bowl, combine the dry ingredients, mixing well one at a time. Once they are thoroughly mixed together, add in the wet ingredients, also thoroughly blending after you add in each ingredient.

Continue to mix as a dough forms. Once it is the right consistency, take a spoon and place rounded cookies on each cookie sheet about 2 inches apart per row.

Only make 2 rows.

Place in the oven and bake for 8 – 10 minutes.

Remove from oven and place on rack to cool.

Gone Nutty

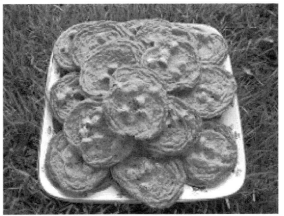

Photo made by: starathena

Makes: 24

Calories: 45

Carbs: 2g

Fats: 3g

What you will need:

½ cup nut butter of your choice

2 tsp almond oil

2 eggs

½ teaspoon vanilla extract

1 teaspoon cinnamon

1 tablespoon coconut flour

¼ cup chopped pecans

1 cup coconut

Directions:

Preheat oven to 350 degrees F.

Spray 2 cookie sheets with no stick cooking spray, or line with parchment paper and set aside.

You are going to use 2 different bowls. Combine all the wet ingredients in one bowl, and all the dry ingredients in another. Slowly add the wet ingredients to the dry ingredients, mixing the entire time.

Continue to mix as a dough forms. Once it is the right consistency, take a spoon and place rounded cookies on each cookie sheet about 2 inches apart per row.

Only make 2 rows.

Place in the oven and bake 12 – 14 minutes.

Remove from oven and place on rack to cool.

Bacon Busters

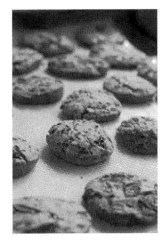

Photo made by: dgbury

Makes: 12

Calories: 66

Carbs: 3g

Fats: 5g

What you will need:

slices bacon, cooked crisp and crumbled

1 cup peanut butter

1 cup granular Stevia

1 large egg

1/2 cup unsweetened organic cocoa powder

1 1/2 tsp vanilla extract

1 tsp baking soda

Directions:

Preheat oven to 350 degrees F. Make sure you start with cooked bacon!

Spray 2 cookie sheets with no stick cooking spray, or line with parchment paper and set aside.

In a large bowl, combine the dry ingredients, mixing well one at a time. Once they are thoroughly mixed together, add in the wet ingredients, also thoroughly blending after you add in each ingredient.

Continue to mix as a dough forms. Once it is the right consistency, take a spoon and place rounded cookies on each cookie sheet about 2 inches apart per row.

Only make 2 rows.

Place in the oven and bake 10 minutes.

Remove from oven and place on rack to cool.

Almond Joys

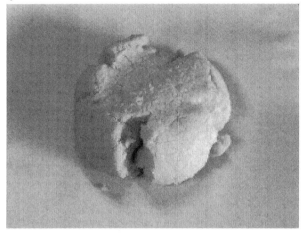

Makes: 42

Calories: 35

Carbs: 1.3g

Fats: 2g

What you will need:

½ Cup of Butter, softened

⅔ Cup of Sweetener

⅔ Cup of Ricotta Cheese

2 Cups of Almond Flour

2 Teaspoons of Vanilla Extract

1 Teaspoon of Almond Extract

1½ Teaspoons of Baking Powder

1 Egg

Directions:

Preheat oven to 350 degrees F.

Spray 2 cookie sheets with no stick cooking spray, or line with parchment paper and set aside.

In a large bowl, combine the dry ingredients, mixing well one at a time. Once they are thoroughly mixed together, add in the wet ingredients, also thoroughly blending after you add in each ingredient.

Continue to mix as a dough forms. Once it is the right consistency, take a spoon and place rounded cookies on each cookie sheet about 2 inches apart per row.

Only make 2 rows.

Place in the oven and bake 15 minutes.

Remove from oven and place on rack to cool.

Lying on a Beach

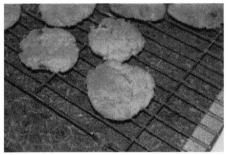

Makes: 18

Calories: 27

Carbs: 2g

Fats: 3g

What you will need:

2 Tbsp almond butter

1 Tbsp coconut oil

1/4 cup coconut milk

2 Tbsp coconut syrup

2 large eggs

1/2 tsp baking powder

1/2 tsp salt

2 Tbsp granulated sugar substitute

1 1/2 cups dried coconut flakes

1/2 cup flax meal

2 squares dark chocolate

¼ cup almonds

Directions:

Preheat oven to 375 degrees F.

Spray 2 cookie sheets with no stick cooking spray, or line with parchment paper and set aside.

You are going to use 2 different bowls. Combine all the wet ingredients in one bowl, and all the dry ingredients in another. Slowly add the wet ingredients to the dry ingredients, mixing the entire time.

Continue to mix as a dough forms. Once it is the right consistency, take a spoon and place rounded cookies on each cookie sheet about 2 inches apart per row.

Only make 2 rows.

Place in the oven and bake 20 minutes.

Remove from oven and place on rack to cool.

Cinnamon Snaps

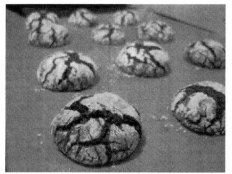

Photo made by: cristinabe

Makes: 18

Calories: 36

Carbs: 2g

Fats: 2g

What you will need:

1 stick butter

¼ cup honey

1 Tbsp vanilla

½ teaspoons salt

¼ teaspoon baking powder

Pinch of cinnamon

Directions:

Preheat oven to 350 degrees F.

Spray 2 cookie sheets with no stick cooking spray, or line with parchment paper and set aside.

In a large bowl, combine the dry ingredients, mixing well one at a time. Once they are thoroughly mixed together, add in the wet ingredients, also thoroughly blending after you add in each ingredient.

Continue to mix as a dough forms. Once it is the right consistency, take a spoon and place rounded cookies on each cookie sheet about 2 inches apart per row.

Only make 2 rows. Place in the oven and bake 8-12 minutes.

Remove from oven and place on rack to cool.

Chunky Chocolate Munchies

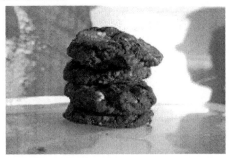

Photo made by: mastermaq

Makes: 20

Calories: 25

Carbs: 1g

Fats: 3g

What you will need:

1 stick unsalted room temperature butter

1 tsp vanilla extract

1/4 cup applesauce,

2 cups almond flour

3 Tbsp cocoa powder

1/4 tsp + 1/8 tsp stevia

1/2 tsp salt

Directions:

Preheat oven to 300 degrees F.

Spray 2 cookie sheets with no stick cooking spray, or line with parchment paper and set aside.

You are going to use 2 different bowls. Combine all the wet ingredients in one bowl, and all the dry ingredients in another. Slowly add the wet ingredients to the dry ingredients, mixing the entire time.

Continue to mix as a dough forms. Once it is the right consistency, take a spoon and place rounded cookies on each cookie sheet about 2 inches apart per row.

Only make 2 rows.

Place in the oven and bake 35 minutes.

Remove from oven and place on rack to cool.

Bites of Heaven

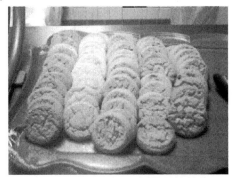

Photo made by: verafevi

Makes: 12

Calories: 42

Carbs: 3g

Fats: 2g

What you will need:

1 cup peanut butter

1 cup erythritol

1 teaspoon sugar free sweetener of your choice

1 egg

1 teaspoon vanilla

1/2 teaspoon salt

Directions:

Preheat oven to 350 degrees F.

Spray 2 cookie sheets with no stick cooking spray, or line with parchment paper and set aside.

You are going to use 2 different bowls. Combine all the wet ingredients in one bowl, and all the dry ingredients in another. Slowly add the wet ingredients to the dry ingredients, mixing the entire time.

Continue to mix as a dough forms. Once it is the right consistency, take a spoon and place rounded cookies on each cookie sheet about 2 inches apart per row.

Only make 2 rows.

Place in the oven and bake 10 minutes.

Remove from oven and place on rack to cool.

Power to the Peanut

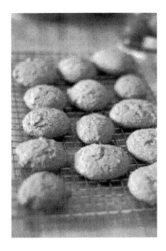

Photo made by: izik

Makes: 60

Calories: 117

Carbs: 4g

Fats: 15g

What you will need:

1 1/2 cups almond flour

1 cup peanut flour

3 tbsp coconut flour

1 tsp baking powder

1/2 tsp salt

1 cup peanut butter

3/4 cup butter, softened

1 cup stevia

2 eggs

1 tsp vanilla

1/4 cup stevia

Directions:

Preheat oven to 325 degrees F.

Spray 2 cookie sheets with no stick cooking spray, or line with parchment paper and set aside.

You are going to use 2 different bowls. Combine all the wet ingredients in one bowl, and all the dry ingredients in another. Slowly add the wet ingredients to the dry ingredients, mixing the entire time.

Continue to mix as a dough forms. Once it is the right consistency, take a spoon and place rounded cookies on each cookie sheet about 2 inches apart per row.

Only make 2 rows.

Place in the oven and bake 10 minutes.

Remove from oven and place on rack to cool.

Minty Magic

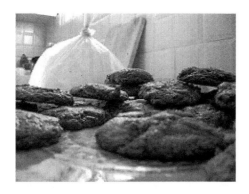

Makes: 40

Calories: 93

Carbs: 2.18g

Fats: 13g

What you will need:

1 3/4 cups coconut flour

1/3 cup cocoa powder

1/4 cup stevia

1 tsp baking powder

1/4 tsp salt

1 large egg, slightly beaten

2 tbsp butter, melted

1/2 teaspoon vanilla extract

1/8 teaspoon stevia

2 tablespoons mint extract

Directions:

Preheat oven to 300 degrees F.

Spray 2 cookie sheets with no stick cooking spray, or line with parchment paper and set aside.

In a large bowl, combine the dry ingredients, mixing well one at a time. Once they are thoroughly mixed together, add in the wet ingredients, also thoroughly blending after you add in each ingredient.

Continue to mix as a dough forms. Once it is the right consistency, take a spoon and place rounded cookies on each cookie sheet about 2 inches apart per row.

Only make 2 rows.

Place in the oven and bake at 15 minutes.

Remove from oven and place on rack to cool.

Somethin' Pumpkin

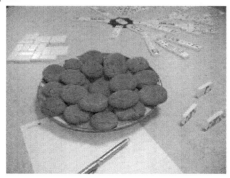

Photo made by: Brian Turner

Makes: 36

Calories: 89

Carbs: 3g

Fats: 9g

What you will need:

3/4 cup honey

3/4 cup canned pumpkin

1/2 cup butter, melted

1 Tbsp vanilla

1 egg

1/2 cup coconut flour

1 1/2 teaspoon cinnamon

1/2 teaspoon sea salt

1/2 teaspoon baking soda

1/2 teaspoon nutmeg

1/4 teaspoon ground cloves

1/4 teaspoon ginger
1 cup semi-sweet chocolate chips

Directions:
Preheat oven to 350 degrees F.

Spray 2 cookie sheets with no stick cooking spray, or line with parchment paper and set aside.

You are going to use 2 different bowls. Combine all the wet ingredients in one bowl, and all the dry ingredients in another. Slowly add the wet ingredients to the dry ingredients, mixing the entire time.

Continue to mix as a dough forms. Once it is the right consistency, take a spoon and place rounded cookies on each cookie sheet about 2 inches apart per row.

Only make 2 rows.

Place in the oven and bake 10 – 15 minutes.

Remove from oven and place on rack to cool.

Perfectly Pumpkin for All

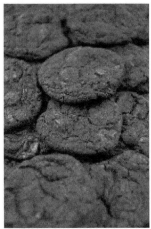

Photo made by: sk8geek

Makes: 24

Calories: 66

Carbs: 3.16g

Fats: 2g

What you will need:

¾ cups canned pumpkin

2 teaspoons coconut oil

2 eggs

½ teaspoon vanilla extract

1 teaspoon ground cinnamon

1 cup coconut

1 Tbsp coconut flour

Directions:

Preheat oven to 350 degrees F.

Spray 2 cookie sheets with no stick cooking spray, or line with parchment paper and set aside.

In a large bowl, combine the dry ingredients, mixing well one at a time. Once they are thoroughly mixed together, add in the wet ingredients, also thoroughly blending after you add in each ingredient.

Continue to mix as a dough forms. Once it is the right consistency, take a spoon and place rounded cookies on each cookie sheet about 2 inches apart per row.

Only make 2 rows.

Place in the oven and bake 15 minutes.

Remove from oven and place on rack to cool.

Pumpkin Doodles

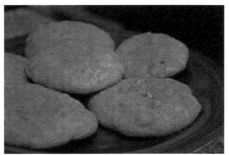

Photo made by: sometoast

Makes: 15

Calories: 104

Carbs: 2.99g

Fats: 1.3g

What you will need:

1 ½ cups almond flour

¼ cup salted butter

½ cup canned pumpkin

1 teaspoon vanilla extract

½ teaspoon baking powder

1 large egg

¼ cup erythritol

25 drops Stevia

73

Directions:

Preheat oven to 350 degrees F.

Spray 2 cookie sheets with no stick cooking spray, or line with parchment paper and set aside.

You are going to use 2 different bowls. Combine all the wet ingredients in one bowl, and all the dry ingredients in another. Slowly add the wet ingredients to the dry ingredients, mixing the entire time.

Continue to mix as a dough forms. Once it is the right consistency, take a spoon and place rounded cookies on each cookie sheet about 2 inches apart per row.

Only make 2 rows.

Place in the oven and bake 10 minutes.

Remove from oven and place on rack to cool.

Crunchinators

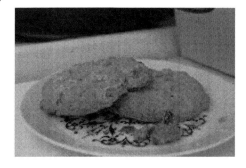

Photo made by: stuart_spivack

Makes: 12

Calories: 64

Carbs: 1.69g

Fats: 6.12g

What you will need:

1/4 cup butter

1/3 cup Stevia

2 tsp molasses

1/4 tsp xanthan gum

1/4 cup Bob's Red Mill almond meal

6 Tbsp Bob's Red Mill coconut

1/2 teaspoon vanilla extract

Directions:

Preheat oven to 350 degrees F.

Spray 2 cookie sheets with no stick cooking spray, or line with parchment paper and set aside.

In a large bowl, combine the dry ingredients, mixing well one at a time. Once they are thoroughly mixed together, add in the wet ingredients, also thoroughly blending after you add in each ingredient.

Continue to mix as a dough forms. Once it is the right consistency, take a spoon and place rounded cookies on each cookie sheet about 2 inches apart per row.

Only make 2 rows.

Place in the oven and bake 12 minutes.

Remove from oven and place on rack to cool.

Now That's Peanut Butter Cookies

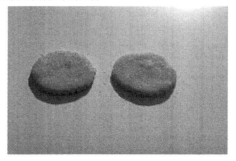

Photo made by: stuart_spivack

Makes: 18

Calories: 67

Carbs: 3.14g

Fats: 4g

What you will need:

1 cup peanut butter

1 1/3 cup Splenda

1 egg

1 teaspoon vanilla

Directions:

Preheat oven to 350 degrees F.

Spray 2 cookie sheets with no stick cooking spray, or line with parchment paper and set aside.

You are going to use 2 different bowls. Combine all the wet ingredients in one bowl, and all the dry ingredients in another. Slowly add the wet ingredients to the dry ingredients, mixing the entire time.

Continue to mix as a dough forms. Once it is the right consistency, take a spoon and place rounded cookies on each cookie sheet about 2 inches apart per row.

Only make 2 rows.

Place in the oven and bake 12 minutes.

Remove from oven and place on rack to cool.

All About that Almond

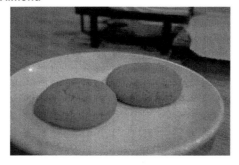

Makes: 18

Calories: 78

Carbs: 3g

Fats: 4g

What you will need:

1 cup crunchy almond butter

1 1/3 cup Splenda

1 egg

1 teaspoon vanilla

Directions:

Preheat oven to 350 degrees F.

Spray 2 cookie sheets with no stick cooking spray, or line with parchment paper and set aside.

In a large bowl, combine the dry ingredients, mixing well one at a time. Once they are thoroughly mixed together, add in the wet ingredients, also thoroughly blending after you add in each ingredient.

Continue to mix as a dough forms. Once it is the right consistency, take a spoon and place rounded cookies on each cookie sheet about 2 inches apart per row.

Only make 2 rows.

Place in the oven and bake 12 – 15 minutes.

Remove from oven and place on rack to cool.

That's What I'm Talking About

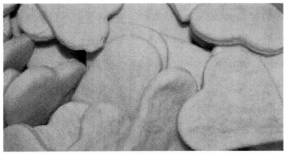

Photo made by: michaelpollak

Makes: 30

Calories: 116

Carbs: 4g

Fats: 11g

What you will need:

¼ cup coconut flour

2 scoops vanilla protein powder
¾ teaspoons baking powder
½ teaspoons xanthan gum
¼ teaspoons salt
1 Tbsp chia seeds
1 Tbsp lemon zest
1 ½ Tbsp coconut oil
1 large egg, room temperature
1 teaspoons vanilla extract
3 Tbsp freshly squeezed lemon juice
¼ cups agave
2 Tbsp Stevia
2 Tbsp Truvia
Directions:

Preheat oven to 325 degrees F.

Spray 2 cookie sheets with no stick cooking spray, or line with parchment paper and set aside.

You are going to use 2 different bowls. Combine all the wet ingredients in one bowl, and all the dry ingredients in another. Slowly add the wet ingredients to the dry ingredients, mixing the entire time.

Continue to mix as a dough forms. Once it is the right consistency, take a spoon and place rounded cookies on each cookie sheet about 2 inches apart per row.

Only make 2 rows.

Place in the oven and bake 11-13 minutes.

Remove from oven and place on rack to cool.

PB and J Delights

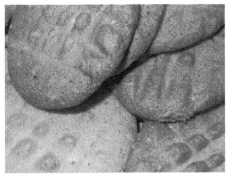

Photo made by: sarahakabmg

Makes: 20

Calories: 158

Carbs: 6g

Fats: 12g

What you will need:

1 3/4 cup sugar free peanut butter

2 eggs

2 Tbsp coconut flour

1 tsp vanilla extract

1/2 tsp baking powder

1 1/3 cup Stevia

1/4 cup sugar free strawberry preserves

Directions:

Preheat oven to 350 degrees F.

Spray 2 cookie sheets with no stick cooking spray, or line with parchment paper and set aside.

In a large bowl, combine the dry ingredients, mixing well one at a time. Once they are thoroughly mixed together, add in the wet ingredients, also thoroughly blending after you add in each ingredient.

Continue to mix as a dough forms. Once it is the right consistency, take a spoon and place rounded cookies on each cookie sheet about 2 inches apart per row.

Only make 2 rows.

Place in the oven and bake 11 minutes.

Remove from oven and place on rack to cool.

Chocolate Meets Peanut Butter

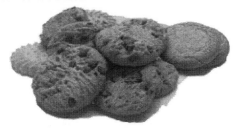

Photo made by: whealie

Makes: 18

Calories: 92

Carbs: 4g

Fats: 8.2g

What you will need:

1 cup peanut butter

1 1/3 cup Splenda

1 egg

1 teaspoon vanilla

½ cup mini chocolate chips

Directions:

Preheat oven to 350 degrees F.

Spray 2 cookie sheets with no stick cooking spray, or line with parchment paper and set aside.

You are going to use 2 different bowls. Combine all the wet ingredients in one bowl, and all the dry ingredients in another. Slowly add the wet ingredients to the dry ingredients, mixing the entire time.

Continue to mix as a dough forms. Once it is the right consistency, take a spoon and place rounded cookies on each cookie sheet about 2 inches apart per row.

Only make 2 rows.

Place in the oven and bake 10 – 12 minutes.

Remove from oven and place on rack to cool.

Snickerdoodles with a Twist

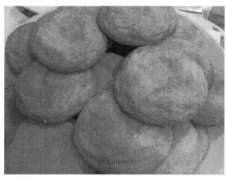

Photo made by: verybadlady

Makes: 24

Calories: 116

Carbs: 5g

Fats: 3.11g

What you will need:

1 ½ cups coconut flour

¼ cup salted butter

½ cup applesauce

1 teaspoon vanilla extract

½ teaspoon baking powder

1 large egg

¼ cup erythritol

25 drops sugar substitute of choice

Directions:

Preheat oven to

Spray 2 cookie sheets with no stick cooking spray, or line with parchment paper and set aside.

In a large bowl, combine the dry ingredients, mixing well one at a time. Once they are thoroughly mixed together, add in the wet ingredients, also thoroughly blending after you add in each ingredient.

Continue to mix as a dough forms. Once it is the right consistency, take a spoon and place rounded cookies on each cookie sheet about 2 inches apart per row.

Only make 2 rows.

Place in the oven and bake at

Remove from oven and place on rack to cool.

Shout Out to Shortbread

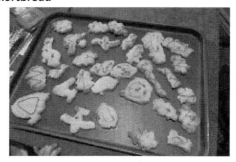

Photo made by: acme

Makes: 24

Calories: 236

Carbs: 3g

Fats: 21g

What you will need:

2 cups coconut flour

1/2 tsp baking powder

1/2 cup butter, softened

1/2 cup Stevia

1 egg yolk

1/2 teaspoon vanilla extract

Directions:

Preheat oven to 325 degrees F.

Spray 2 cookie sheets with no stick cooking spray, or line with parchment paper and set aside.

In a large bowl, combine the dry ingredients, mixing well one at a time. Once they are thoroughly mixed together, add in the wet ingredients, also thoroughly blending after you add in each ingredient.

Continue to mix as a dough forms. Once it is the right consistency, take a spoon and place rounded cookies on each cookie sheet about 2 inches apart per row.

Only make 2 rows.

Place in the oven and bake 14 minutes.

Remove from oven and place on rack to cool.

Chocolate on Chocolate

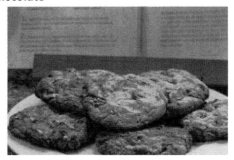

Photo made by: Jim Lukach

Makes: 24

Calories: 166

Carbs: 3.42g

Fats: 11g

What you will need:

1 3/4 cups coconut flour

1/3 cup cocoa powder

1/4 cup stevia

1 tsp baking powder

1/4 tsp salt

1 large egg, slightly beaten

2 tbsp butter, melted

1/2 teaspoon vanilla extract

½ cup unsweetened chocolate chips

Directions:

Preheat oven to 350 degrees F.

Spray 2 cookie sheets with no stick cooking spray, or line with parchment paper and set aside.

You are going to use 2 different bowls. Combine all the wet ingredients in one bowl, and all the dry ingredients in another. Slowly add the wet ingredients to the dry ingredients, mixing the entire time.

Continue to mix as a dough forms. Once it is the right consistency, take a spoon and place rounded cookies on each cookie sheet about 2 inches apart per row.

Only make 2 rows.

Place in the oven and bake 10 – 12 minutes.

Remove from oven and place on rack to cool.

All That Jazz

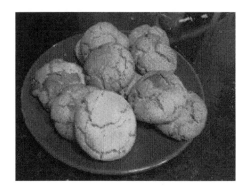

Photo made by: kalleboo

Makes: 24

Calories: 118

Carbs: 4g

Fats: 9g

What you will need:

1 1/2 cups almond flour

1/2 cup cocoa powder

1/2 teaspoon baking soda

1/2 teaspoon salt

1/2 cup Stevia

1/2 cup butter, cut into small pieces

2 large eggs

1 teaspoon vanilla extract

5 1/2 ounces chocolate

Directions:

Preheat oven to 325 degrees F.

Spray 2 cookie sheets with no stick cooking spray, or line with parchment paper and set aside.

In a large bowl, combine the dry ingredients, mixing well one at a time. Once they are thoroughly mixed together, add in the wet ingredients, also thoroughly blending after you add in each ingredient.

Continue to mix as a dough forms. Once it is the right consistency, take a spoon and place rounded cookies on each cookie sheet about 2 inches apart per row.

Only make 2 rows.

Place in the oven and bake

Remove from oven and place on rack to cool.

Sunday Strawberry Shortcake Cookies

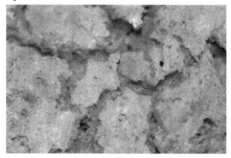

Photo made by: ahuett

Makes: 24

Calories: 244

Carbs: 4g

Fats: 13g

What you will need:

2 cups almond flour

1/3 cup strawberry preserves – sugar free

1/2 tsp baking powder

1/2 cup butter, softened

1/2 cup Stevia

1 egg yolk

1/2 teaspoon vanilla extract

Directions:

Preheat oven to 325 degrees F.

Spray 2 cookie sheets with no stick cooking spray, or line with parchment paper and set aside.

You are going to use 2 different bowls. Combine all the wet ingredients in one bowl, and all the dry ingredients in another. Slowly add the wet ingredients to the dry ingredients, mixing the entire time.

Continue to mix as a dough forms. Once it is the right consistency, take a spoon and place rounded cookies on each cookie sheet about 2 inches apart per row.

Only make 2 rows.

Place in the oven and bake 12-14 minutes.

Remove from oven and place on rack to cool.

Power Balls

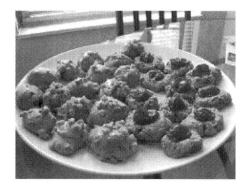

Photo made by: kinggrl

Makes: 6

Calories: 56

Carbs: 5.6g

Fats: 1.8g

What you will need:

1 Tbsp peanut butter

1/3 cup dry oatmeal

1 package sugar free hot cocoa mix

¼ teaspoon baking powder

½ scoop whey protein powder

2 packets Stevia

Directions:

Preheat oven to 300 degrees F.

Spray 2 cookie sheets with no stick cooking spray, or line with parchment paper and set aside.

In a large bowl, combine the dry ingredients, mixing well one at a time. Once they are thoroughly mixed together, add in the wet ingredients, also thoroughly blending after you add in each ingredient.

Continue to mix as a dough forms. Once it is the right consistency, take a spoon and place rounded cookies on each cookie sheet about 2 inches apart per row.

Only make 2 rows.

Place in the oven and bake 10 minutes.

Remove from oven and place on rack to cool.

Fall Fashion Cookies

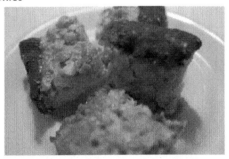

Photo made by: mfoetsch

95

Makes: 26

Calories: 40

Carbs: 3g

Fats: 2g

What you will need:

1/4 cup ground flax seed,

2 Tbsp chia seeds

1/2 Tbsp of ground cinnamon

3 large eggs

2 teaspoons vanilla

1/4 cup of light almond milk

1/4 cup Stevia in the raw

2 servings whey protein powder

1 teaspoon baking soda

1 teaspoon baking powder

1 can pumpkin

Directions:

Preheat oven to 350 degrees.

Spray 2 cookie sheets with no stick cooking spray, or line with parchment paper and set aside.

You are going to use 2 different bowls. Combine all the wet ingredients in one bowl, and all the dry ingredients in another. Slowly add the wet ingredients to the dry ingredients, mixing the entire time.

Continue to mix as a dough forms. Once it is the right consistency, take a spoon and place rounded cookies on each cookie sheet about 2 inches apart per row.

Only make 2 rows.

Place in the oven and bake 10 – 12 minutes.

Remove from oven and place on rack to cool.

Better Than Butter Cookies

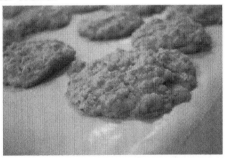

Photo made by: slgc

Makes: 28

Calories: 149

Carbs: 5.3g

Fats: 4g

What you will need:

2 sticks butter

2 Tbsp water

¾ cup sugar free sweetener of choice

2 eggs

½ teaspoons vanilla

½ cup sugar free brown sugar substitute

1 cup almond flour

1/3 cup coconut flour

1 teaspoons baking soda

½ teaspoon baking powder

¼ teaspoon salt

4 cups flaked coconut

Directions:

Preheat oven to 350 degrees F.

Spray 2 cookie sheets with no stick cooking spray, or line with parchment paper and set aside.

In a large bowl, combine the dry ingredients, mixing well one at a time. Once they are thoroughly mixed together, add in the wet ingredients, also thoroughly blending after you add in each ingredient.

Continue to mix as a dough forms. Once it is the right consistency, take a spoon and place rounded cookies on each cookie sheet about 2 inches apart per row.

Only make 2 rows.

Place in the oven and bake 8 – 10 minutes.

Remove from oven and place on rack to cool.

Mad Munchies

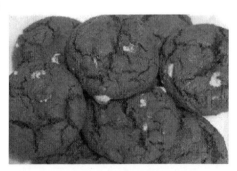

Photo made by: jamiejamison

Makes: 18

Calories: 112

Carbs: 4.4g

Fats: 4g

What you will need:

2 1/2 cup almond flour

1/2 tsp salt

1/2 tsp baking soda

1/2 cup coconut oil

1 Tbsp vanilla extract

1/2 cup powdered erythritol

1/2 cup dark chocolate chips

1/4 chopped walnuts

Directions:

Preheat oven to 350 degrees F.

Spray 2 cookie sheets with no stick cooking spray, or line with parchment paper and set aside.

In a large bowl, combine the dry ingredients, mixing well one at a time. Once they are thoroughly mixed together, add in the wet ingredients, also thoroughly blending after you add in each ingredient.

Continue to mix as a dough forms. Once it is the right consistency, take a spoon and place rounded cookies on each cookie sheet about 2 inches apart per row.

Only make 2 rows.

Place in the oven and bake 10 – 12 minutes.

Remove from oven and place on rack to cool.

Best Ever Chocolate Chip Cookies

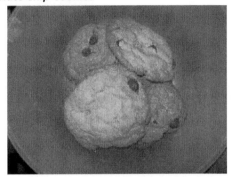

Photo made by: drummerchick

Makes: 18

Calories: 133

Carbs: 4g

Fats: 3.11g

What you will need:

3 eggs

1⁄2 cup softened butter

1 teaspoon vanilla extract

1⁄2 teaspoon cinnamon

1⁄2 teaspoon nutmeg

2 teaspoons stevia

1⁄3 cup coconut flour

1⁄2 teaspoon baking soda

1⁄2 teaspoon sea salt

1 cup almond meal

4-6 ounce unsweetened dark chocolate

Directions:

Preheat oven to 350 degrees F.

Spray 2 cookie sheets with no stick cooking spray, or line with parchment paper and set aside.

You are going to use 2 different bowls. Combine all the wet ingredients in one bowl, and all the dry ingredients in another. Slowly add the wet ingredients to the dry ingredients, mixing the entire time.

Continue to mix as a dough forms. Once it is the right consistency, take a spoon and place rounded cookies on each cookie sheet about 2 inches apart per row.

Only make 2 rows.

Place in the oven and bake 15 minutes.

Remove from oven and place on rack to cool.

Nut Attack

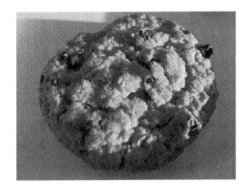

Photo made by: glennf

Makes: 30

Calories: 165

Carbs: 5g

Fats: 3g

What you will need:

1 3/4 cups almond flour

1/3 cup cocoa powder

1/4 cup stevia

1 tsp baking powder

1/4 teaspoon salt

1 large egg, slightly beaten

2 tbsp butter, melted

1/2 teaspoon vanilla extract

¼ cup crunchy almond butter

½ cup chopped almonds

Directions:

Preheat oven to 350 degrees F.

Spray 2 cookie sheets with no stick cooking spray, or line with parchment paper and set aside.

In a large bowl, combine the dry ingredients, mixing well one at a time. Once they are thoroughly mixed together, add in the wet ingredients, also thoroughly blending after you add in each ingredient.

Continue to mix as a dough forms. Once it is the right consistency, take a spoon and place rounded cookies on each cookie sheet about 2 inches apart per row.

Only make 2 rows.

Place in the oven and bake 12-14 minutes.

Remove from oven and place on rack to cool.

Conclusion

There you have it, 30 recipes that will give you your sweet satisfaction while sticking with your low carb goals. These cookies are perfect for those moments when you need something sweet but don't want to break your diet, and they are going to help you reach your goals faster than ever.

The results are real, the cookies are amazing, and they have never been easier to make. You are going to fall in love with each and every one of these recipes – and you are going to love the number on the scale each time you step on.

Get ready to drop those pant sizes, because you really can have your cookies and eat them, too.

27690634R00059

Printed in Great Britain
by Amazon